Surviving Dementia Without Losing Your Mind

*The Essential Home Care Guide
For Families and Caregivers*

MARISA PASQUINI

Surviving Dementia Without Losing Your Mind:
The Essential Home Care Guide for Families and Caregivers

Published by
National Home Care Academy Press
Santa Barbara, CA 93105

survivingdementiabook.com

Paperback: 978-1-64184-800-8

Cover Design: Melodee Meyer
Photo of Marisa Pasquini: Madeleine Vite

Printed and Manufactured in the United States of America.

Dear Reader,

I'm so glad you're reading this book because it tells me that you care about someone with dementia, and I'm here to support you.

I hope you find useful tools in the pages to follow. There are other free resources included with this book. You can find them at:

survivingdementiabook.com

Connect with me! I'd love to hear from you.

Peace and Joy,
Marisa

For Olivia and Rachael.

Anything is possible.

TABLE OF CONTENTS

INTRODUCTION

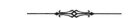

I met Kerry a year after her diagnosis with early-onset Alzheimer's. She was 47 years old. I was hired as Kerry's "driver," a pseudonym for "caregiver" because Kerry was in complete denial of her disease. She wanted a helper who was close to her in age so she would look good in public, like two girls hanging out. She would knock anyone to their knees with cutting remarks if they dare insinuate that she needed help of any kind.

By the time I met her, Kerry already had some great strategies to keep up the facade and preserve her image as a "normal" person. She had key phrases that she repeated: "Never bored," she'd smile. "Gotta keep moving!" and even, "It's so good to see you!" She was great at pretending that she was ok and that was how she liked it.

Kerry was an outstanding athlete and played tennis several times a week. She was fit and bright and lovely.

On a sunny day in January, Kerry and I took our first drive to the tennis club. I was so afraid I would put her on the spot somehow, that I'd ask the wrong question and embarrass her. She casually commented on cars that passed by and read street signs while I was a nervous wreck! We had just met and I wanted to connect with her, but I also wasn't sure what she remembered or whether she even liked to talk. I took a deep breath and simply asked, "Have you been playing tennis for a long time?"

Well, I got the answer to my question. Yes, Kerry liked to talk, and she loved talking about tennis.

She turned toward me and beamed. Her face lit up like a Christmas tree! She effervesced about playing tennis since she was "a tiny tot" with her parents. She had played in school and had won a big tournament as a teen. In fact, she was still playing "with all the pros" she said proudly and with a twinkle in her eye. "I hit 'em. I hit 'em hard!" she laughed.

I knew in that moment that we were going to be ok together and that we would be great friends. I couldn't help but love Kerry.

There were many sides to Kerry: strong and athletic, witty, hilarious, and smart as a whip, but she could also be mean, berating and self-loathing.

One day I was putting away some laundry and I accidentally brushed against her as I passed. She nearly jumped out of her skin and savagely fumed at me, "Ouch! Watch what you're doing!" She sneered at me and rubbed her arm as if she'd been burned. Her overreaction was punctuated with pure disgust in her eyes.

We ate lunch together every day. One day I made the mistake of ordering something that she disapproved of. She sneered with insults, calling me a "big gal" and a "butterball."

Many days, she looked me straight in the eyes and dismissively said, "I just need a better helper, someone who will really help me."

She had horrendous meltdowns, raging against herself saying things like, "I'm stupid! I'm useless! I can't even drive! Just throw me out! Put me away! Get away from me. Leave me alone. I'm gonna run. I can run fast, and I'll be gone!"

Her frustration and anger grew to a point where she was violent with her elderly father, who provided night shift care for her. She got angry one night and pushed him, nearly knocking him down. Her outbursts became more and more frequent. It was excruciating to watch her unraveling, especially knowing this hateful behavior stemmed from the pain she was in.

It got to the point that I thought I was losing my mind. I would drive home at the end of the day and literally scream in my car. There were moments when I wanted to run, as fast as I could, and be gone. And there were many moments when I knew I was making a difference for her. I found myself thinking about her and talking about her all the time. The truth was, I didn't want to leave her. I wanted to learn how to be with her and how to really help her.

I talked with social workers, Alzheimer's experts, psychiatrists, and other caregivers. I joined support groups. I read books and blogs and joined online networks. I took notes and recorded conversations. I kept trying and I didn't give up. By listening and implementing the strategies I learned, it changed everything. Everything.

I developed a simple system. It takes a little time to internalize, but once you get it, you find out that life with someone with dementia can be sweet. Yes, I said sweet.

All the caregivers I train and have talked to in writing this book do it for one reason: they care. They want to make a difference for another human being. Me too.

I was eager to give Kerry the best care (and life) possible and to give her family a sense of peace and calm. I was motivated to do things differently than I had done before with her. I became the Kerry Expert.

I created some simple communication techniques and changed the way I interacted with and spoke to her, down to the actual words and phrases I used. As my communication changed, she changed. Her behavior changed. She became less anxious. She had fewer and fewer meltdowns. We joyfully spent many hours together every day, week after week. Best of friends.

Remember how Kerry didn't like to be touched? How she would flinch so hard the floor would shake if you even brushed against her? You won't believe what happened.

Kerry's extreme sensitivities were not only to touch, but also to smells, sounds, tastes and textures. All of these are strong triggers for her and I could write volumes on each of them! At one point, she decided that she couldn't go to the "hairdo parlor" anymore because it was too stinky. Yet, she wanted her hair colored.

I had been taking care of Kerry's nails for a while, so *she* suggested that we buy color and I apply it for her. Considering her sensitivities and her raging, I was skeptical as to how successful this would be, but I played along.

We entered the beauty supply shop and looked at the rows and rows of potions and products. We picked some hair color with the help of a purple-haired girl who enthusiastically plucked items off shelves for us. Kerry was like a kid in a candy store! Then we headed home to sample our wares.

I mixed the product and draped her with an old towel. She sat down comfortably on a chair in her kitchen, closed her eyes, and let me brush on the color. I moved slowly and methodically and she relaxed completely. It was like watching someone in a meditative state. She breathed softly and had a little smile on her face. I felt like a hero.

That anxious, irritable person completely relaxed in my presence. It was a truly pivotal moment for me. I knew that she trusted me and felt safe with me and that she was different. It was then that I knew I was onto something. I knew that I had to share this information with others who were caring for people with dementia.

In this book, I share my methods with you. These are tips and strategies that are tried and true by me and many other successful, happy caregivers. We're happy because our loved ones are happy.

CHAPTER 1

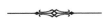

What Is Happening Here?

Jane: Hi Mom, is Dad there?

Mom: Yes, dear, hold on just a minute. I'll put him on.

        (Dad gets on the phone)

Jane: Dad, I wanted to let you know that I'm…

Dad: (interrupts) There's a show on TV about Italy.

        Do you want to watch it?

Jane: Um…I'm not there, Dad. I'm in Iowa.

Dad: What are you doing there?

Jane: Dad, I live here. I want to talk to you about…

Dad: Hold on, I'll get your mother.

Jane: No. No... Dad?

        (Mom gets on the phone)

Jane: Dad can't seem to focus on what I'm...

Mom: Don't you worry about your Dad. He's fine.
        He's got me.

Jane: Ok, Well, who do you have?

Mom: I have your father. Hang on just a minute,
        I'll put him on.

This scene from a popular TV show hit home for me because it accurately illustrates the situation we find ourselves in as our parents age. We wake up and realize our parents are not who they used to be. They are not just slowing down, they're forgetting important information. They're repeating themselves. What else are they forgetting that we just aren't noticing? It's frightening to think of our parents in this vulnerable situation, especially if we live far away.

According to a report from the Alzheimer's Association, over six million Americans are currently diagnosed with Alzheimer's or another form of dementia. By year 2050, that number is expected to reach 14 million.

Every year,15 million family caregivers provide 18.4 billion hours of care for people with dementia in the United States. The cost of care is valued at over $232 billion.

According the Family Caregiver Alliance, 8,357,000 seniors in the US are making use of some type of long-term care. That number is almost equal to the population of New York City.

Between the years 2000 and 2015, deaths from heart disease decreased by 11% while deaths from Alzheimer's increased 123%.

According to the Alzheimer's Association, dementia-related disease is the sixth leading cause of death in America. It is estimated that one in three seniors die with a form of dementia or Alzheimer's. However, this number may be much higher. *Neurology,* the official journal of the American Academy of Neurology and a leading peer-reviewed journal, reported that "a groundbreaking study from researchers at the Rush Alzheimer's Disease Center in Chicago attributes more than 500,000 deaths (in 2010) to Alzheimer's disease, "which is six times the number reported by the Center for Disease Control in the same time period.

The statistics are staggering. In fact, they're overwhelming, which is the point. Based on these figures, there isn't one of us that will escape the effects of dementia or Alzheimer's within our families or with other loved ones in our lives. When we have a conversation with our mothers or fathers like the one above, we wonder, "Will I be next?"

My friend Mark lives half a continent away from his mother. She started forgetting things: names, dates, when she spoke to him last, and he knew that something had to be done... but how? He cannot be a permanent caregiver for his mother. He lives and works in California and like most adult children, he can't just pick up and move across the country to be a caregiver. But what if a catastrophe happened, a heart attack or stroke or a fall? Would there be someone there who knows her day-to-day routine to be in charge and make sure she gets the care she needs? What if something happens and she can't bounce back?

I met a woman whose father-in-law has Alzheimer's. He moved into her home with her, her husband, and their seven-month-old twins. She's now caregiver to two actual babies and one adult baby.

I have a client whose parents are quite elderly. They are both still very bright and independent. Dad has had several falls and transient ischemic attacks (TIA). Mom is still very active and wants to continue her activities. The children want their dad to be safe and their mom to continue with her interests. The kids want to put something in place for their parents to prepare for the future. They're scared to death that something will happen and then they will have to deal with it on an emergency basis and have fewer choices.

We are afraid because our parents lie or hide their reality from their children and then it will be too late to get help for them. We don't want one parent being overwhelmed with care giving for the other parent. We worry about our parents being taken advantage of, which is another very real fear.

One of my first clients was the mother of my dearest friend Ann. Her lovely mom began wandering, trying to find her dead husband. The day came when police found her and fitted her with a tracking device. I will never forget the look on her face as the officer gently attached the bracelet on her arm. It was simply a look of a failure.

Perhaps the mom who was such an adventurer is now too afraid to get into an elevator. She stays inside her house all day, watching movies and is not really living life. In a sense, she dies before she's even dead.

Parents can be fiercely independent and lie or hide their difficulties from their children. They're caregiving for each other and becoming increasingly overwhelmed, but still not saying anything to anyone about it. Bringing outside caregivers has its own set of issues because we want someone we can trust when we can't be there, people who will respect our parents, their values and their property. We have real fears about our parents being taken advantage of. We want to know that our parents are enjoying their lives, have satisfying activities and companionship, and most of all, that they're safe.

Adult children and families are dealing with caring for their aging parents on all different levels. We're caring for (and financially obligated to) our children and now have the responsibility to care for and pay the costs of caring for our elderly parent or parents. We're looking for the right person to live in our childhood homes. We realize that the essence of our parents is going away. They're a shadow of their former selves. They really are not our parents anymore. We want to come home to Mommy, and we can't...because Mommy is gone.

According to *Psychology Today*, about one out of every eight Americans between the ages of 40 and 60 care directly for an aging parent, and over eight million Americans help their parents or other aging relatives from long distances. These are people with dependent children who need emotional or financial help. The magazine states, "...the number of children caught in this double-bind is expected to grow as more and more members of the baby boom generation become senior citizens themselves." With the hiring situation being more difficult for the younger generation, fewer of them are finding jobs and are living back home with Mom and Dad. It's not surprising that members of the "sandwich generation" feel more and more squeezed and stressed from both sides.

No matter where you are in the process, you are not alone. Help is available whether you are seeing early signs of dementia in your parents or other loved ones, whether you are considering becoming a caregiver yourself or looking for assistance for a loved one. There are ways to continue to have joy during this time of life with your parent or loved one.

Take a breath and read on.

CHAPTER 2

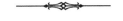

Why I Care

I stepped through the drab and dreary hallways of a skilled nursing facility where my mom was recuperating from a brain bleed caused by a spike in blood pressure. She was just hours out of ICU and was placed in a nearby facility. It was noisy with clanking trays, people calling out from the rooms and staff robotically giving out meds and food.

My mom, eyes closed and mouth open, was sleeping in her narrow bed, covered by a thin blanket. She looked different, smaller. I actually wondered if she was breathing, but, thank God, she was. I softly called out to her, "Hell-ahn" (an old nickname). She cracked a little smile, without even opening her eyes. My heart raced and I thought, "She's in there!! She remembers! She recognizes my voice!"

I knelt beside the bed and continued to speak slowly and softly to her. She finally opened her eyes and looked around. She had absolutely no idea where she was. She was absolutely panicked. She looked like she wanted to get away. Her eyes were wide with fear when she looked at me, her baby. I finally stepped back and asked her gently, "Do you know who I am?" She looked me straight in the eyes and flatly answered, "No."

I was pissed. How could this have happened? I had been out of the country when my Mom had her stroke. I had talked to her once at the beginning of my trip. We were laughing and making plans for when I got back.

She had a stroke the next day.

Standing in line at customs, I turned the cell service back on my phone. After a series of dings, I started reading the texts that were coming in. Texts from my siblings.

"She's still in ICU."

"She hasn't said anything yet. She still can't talk."

"They're keeping her here a few more days."

"I'm leaving in the morning. I'll be there tomorrow."

WTF? I called my brother and he told me the story. I was still across the country and couldn't get home fast enough.

I wasn't ready to lose my mom. I really felt like it was a bad dream, and that someone would nudge me and I'd wake up. When I saw her and she didn't recognize me, I had to face the fact that I might actually lose her in the worst way.

My mom, who is a mother, grandmother, great-grandmother, teacher, friend and advocate, had been shattered. At age 89, she was still living by herself in the house where I was born and raised. She was a faithful Bible reader and teacher. There were six kids in our family. She was the mom who made our lunches every day, the one who had dinner on the table at six o'clock, six nights a week (on Friday's she and my dad had date night). She was the mom who kept score at the bowling alley every week for my brother, Rick (who had intellectual disabilities) and his friends. I felt embarrassed by my brother, and even a little afraid of him and his friends. But not my Mom. She genuinely enjoyed them, and they loved her, too. She sewed clothes for me and did beautiful embroidery work. She held everything together when one of my brothers went missing and was found a week later, drowned under a tree trunk in a rushing river. She tenderly cared for my Dad in 1984 and my brother Rick in 2012, when they each died of cancer. Rick was the same age Dad was when he died.

Mom was called on by our friends when their four-year-old daughter was dying and she was there for her last breath. She's the one who painted so beautifully, winning awards in juried shows. She sang in a choir and could beat the pants off you in a game of Scrabble. She was at the births of my two daughters and never left my side as I became a first-time mother. I remember us trying to bathe my first-born daughter 24 years ago. I was so nervous and afraid I would hurt her and Mom was trying to remember how to do it! We laughed so hard! She helped me through my divorce and empowered me to keep going.

Now the one who was "strong like bull" needed help, needed care. I still wasn't sure how much of her we'd be getting back as the weeks and months went by, or how much worse she might get. I guess my biggest fear was that we wouldn't be so lucky if she had another episode. I braced myself for the worst.

I didn't lose my mom. She is still alive, but she is very much changed. When she has visitors, she is so happy to see them. Then if she turns away and sees them again, it's as if they just arrived! She wants to drive; she can't. She lived alone before this happened and now she needs 24-hour care. She's not sure why she has someone living with her now. "I don't really think I need it..." Thank God my dad made good decisions years ago before he died. Mom has a wonderful caregiver who my siblings and I trust completely.

Mom is at a different stage in her life now, but it doesn't feel bad. Our relationship, conversations and activities are different now, but we still enjoy each other's company. We have plenty of good times that include puzzles and games, drinking coffee, laughing and painting. It's wonderful to see her completely immersed in the moment painting. She is still my mom.

CHAPTER 3

Where Are You?

"Your mom is experiencing some early signs of dementia." When I say it in my head it's almost sing-song. No big deal! Some early signs of dementia! But for a daughter, or spouse or (god forbid) a parent it's life changing. It's funny how all of life can change in just one second and how one short sentence change your entire future. This is what happened to me, to my friends and clients, and probably to you as well. Hearing these terrifying and heartbreaking words fill us with sadness, confusion and panic.

Anyone who has been around it knows that dementia and Alzheimer's are mysterious. The symptoms and declines are unique to each person. While that makes sense as each person's physical makeup, life experiences, personality, beliefs and environment are individual, it also presents genuine problems and questions: How will this dementia progress? Will it turn into full-blown Alzheimer's? How can I prepare? Can I prepare?

There are some behaviors and symptoms that are constant and are outlined in the medical approach to dementia and Alzheimer's. Symptoms and stages can overlap and progression is different for each person. Whether a person you love has received an official diagnosis or you're just noticing signs of memory loss, the overview in this chapter will help you to see where you are and what might be coming as the disease progresses. Knowing the typical stages and declines can help.

OVERVIEW OF ALZHEIMER'S

All dementia is not Alzheimer's, but Alzheimer's is the most common cause of dementia. Dementia is defined as "a group of symptoms affecting memory, thinking and social abilities severely enough to interfere with daily functioning." Alzheimer's disease is the most common cause of dementia. Alzheimer's is framed in seven stages. In the first three stages, a person is not considered to have dementia.

Stage 1: No Impairment

In the first stage, a person with Alzheimer's has no memory impairment and no obvious symptoms of dementia. It's undetectable and sometimes called No Cognitive Decline. This stage can last for 10 or more years and go undetected. There are plans for early diagnosis through testing, to prevent or delay symptoms, but so far trials have been disappointing.

Stage 2: Very Mild Cognitive Decline

In this stage, a person with Alzheimer's disease begins to exhibit the typical forgetfulness we associate with aging such as forgetting where they left keys or a wallet. The symptoms are still not really noticed by family or doctors, except possibly in retrospect. If the person with the memory loss notices, they may cover it up or begin isolating themselves because they don't want anyone to know. If you notice a family member isolating him or herself, you may want to pay a little closer attention.

Stage 3: Mild Cognitive Decline

People in Stage 3 experience increased forgetfulness and lose more ability to focus or concentrate. They may ask the same question they asked just minutes before, forgetting the answer or that they already asked the question. They may become confused about place and time, not knowing where they are or where you are. They may uncharacteristically fixate on a subject or a thing (the plants need to be watered right now!) They struggle to find the right words to express themselves. If they're still in the workforce, their performance will deteriorate. They will lose the ability to organize bills or finances. Stage 3 lasts, on average, about seven years.

Stage 4: Moderate Cognitive Decline

Your doctor will now call the disease or symptoms "dementia."

Stage 4 comprises what is described as Early Stage Dementia. Forgetfulness increases and includes recent events (for instance, they may forget that they saw you just yesterday and wonder why you haven't called or visited). There is increased difficulty problem solving and concentrating. You'll probably want to someone else to handle the finances and your doctor might recommend this. Getting lost in familiar places is typical. No more solo trips to the pharmacy and probably no more driving at this point. A companion is recommended for outings. They may be in denial about their symptoms and memory loss and are probably still trying to hide out. They may get angry if their forgetfulness is exposed. Withdrawal from social activities will increase, even with people they know and love, because socializing and keeping up with conversations becomes more difficult. Depression, paranoia, hoarding, anger, wandering, incontinence and frustration may be seen.

The average duration of Stage 4 is two to 10 years. You will probably notice a decline every four to six months. Finding good medications from a trusted neurologist and psychiatrist will support your loved one as their memory declines.

Stage 5: Moderately Severe Cognitive Decline, Mid-Stage Dementia

At this stage, memory deficits are severe. People at this stage start needing assistance with their daily living: bathing, dressing and preparing meals. They lose track of their words, thoughts and personal history and have difficulty following conversations or understanding what others are trying to communicate. People at this stage typically forget their address, phone number and other prominent bits of information that affect their daily lives. They lose their orientation to place and time. Stage 5 lasts, on average, one to one-and-a-half years.

Stage 6: Severe Cognitive Decline, Middle Dementia

In Stage 6, your loved one now needs considerable care and support to carry out all day-to-day activities. They will have little memory of their earlier life and lose memory of the names of close family, friends, or caregivers. They lose the ability to walk or get themselves up and will start losing language and the ability to speak. People in Stage 6 often, but not always, experience incontinence. Significant personality changes may take place and the person may suffer from anxiety, agitation or delusions. Stage 6, according to medical findings, lasts about two-and-a-half years.

Stage 7: Very Severe Cognitive Decline, Late Stage Dementia

Stage 7, also known as advanced dementia, is the final stage in the progression of Alzheimer's disease. They may think they're in a different time period all together, reverting back to their childhood and mistaking children for siblings or parents or spouses. They may ask to visit long-deceased family or friends. They will eventually have significant issues with communication, often using only words or expressions but not sentences. At the very end, they may not verbally communicate at all and may only use facial expressions. They will require extensive assistance with daily living activities such as personal hygiene and eating. At the very end of this stage, the individual will most likely be bedridden. This severe stage of dementia lasts approximately one to three years.

The bad news is your doctor has about as much an idea as you do as to where your loved one is. I've heard from countless families, and experienced myself, that you're kind of on your own in figuring out what to do and where to go for help when there is someone in your life with dementia. The first two stages of Alzheimer's in the medical model are not even dementia. Stages are not linear, not to mention the normal ups and downs, moods, good days and bad days that accompany the disease. The length of each stage is also questionable because each person experiences symptoms differently. In order to simplify the stages and to assess the needs for care, I describe the "7 Stages" as a three phase system.

CHAPTER 4

The Three Phases of Dementia

We all experience situations where we forget and our first thought is, "Am I getting Alzheimer's?" We see a friend out of context and can't remember his or her name. We lose our keys or phone or forget appointments. It's called the Alzheimer's of overwhelm and we all have it.

I've talked to a lot of people who worry that they have dementia. Smile! If you're worried about it, you probably don't have it. Dementia develops slowly over years and even decades. People with dementia know that it's different than typical forgetfulness and overwhelm. They cover it up. They hide it from family and friends. If they're caught, they might laugh it off, hoping you won't notice, or get really defensive and angry. With dementia, memory loss gets worse and worse over time.

PHASE ONE

Barbara is a good friend of mine. She lives and works in LA. She attended an elite private college, speaks French fluently and considered a career in politics because of her passion for creating change in the world. One day, she strode out of her office on her way to meet a friend for dinner and couldn't remember where she had parked her car. She panicked a little but ended up shrugging her shoulders ultimately laughing about it because of her great sense of humor. She called a friend and told him the situation. He showed up, they searched together, and found where she left the car. They laugh about it and headed off to eat.

We've all experienced something like this, right? Especially with parked cars. We park in some big structure and then forget which floor we parked on. We might take precautions to help us remember when we leave the car. We look at the markers so that we can remember where it is. So, the real problem in Barbara's story isn't that she forgot where she parked her car. The actual problem, and what differentiates signs of dementia from simply forgetting, is that Barbara couldn't retrace her steps. Barbara was diagnosed two years later with early onset Alzheimer's.

This is a classic Phase 1 story. When friends and family members start to see signs of memory loss, it's time to keep a closer watch. Your parent or loved one is still probably doing reasonably well on his or her own, living independently, possibly still working or driving and being socially active. This is the time to take notice and watch from a distance. Barbara carried on with her life independently for several years, and very well, losing cars aside! She was living her life and likely hiding some of her symptoms. This is good news, because she was able to live and function on her own before her diagnosis.

Some families choose to have a helper come in a few hours a week, either a family member, friend or caregiver, as they notice changes. It is a good idea to track any major shifts and also to start learning about the person being cared for. Overall, this is the time to savor the relationship with your loved one, engage in activities that you both enjoy and let them be!

THINGS TO LOOK FOR

Slight lapses in memory

Misplacing items

Isolating

PHASE TWO

A couple of years later, Barbara was showing more symptoms of memory loss. She was still living alone, but her house was bursting with an abundance of paper towels, tissues, mouthwash, dental floss and all kinds of other household items. Her family really wasn't tracking her spending because they had no idea anything was wrong. She was forgetting the Amazon purchases she had just made and kept buying the same things over and over again, day after day. Fortunately, this was harmless spending and with help, she stopped over-buying. She couldn't live alone anymore and so began 24-hour care. This worked well for her for several years until her team couldn't manage her at home anymore.

During Phase 2, you'll be seeing noticeable signs of dementia, mood swings, memory loss and your loved one not functioning well independently. You may find clutter or unpaid bills.

Phase 2 is the longest phase and many changes will take place during this time. You'll start looking for care, making arrangements for assisted living or family caregivers for your loved one throughout Phase 2, but it will start gradually.

By the end of Phase 2, your loved one is going to need a good neurologist who specializes in dementia, a good psychiatrist who can prescribe medication for mood swings or aggression and 24-hour care. Do not despair! There is still a lot of joy to be had!

THINGS TO LOOK FOR

Decreased performance at work or in household management

Issues with organizing or concentrating

Not following conversations

Forgetting recent events

Aggression, Insomnia

PHASE THREE

Barbara finally needed 24-hour care. She was anxious being alone and was moved into assisted living. She was having angry outbursts and her family wanted her to be in a place where she'd have adequate help for the long term. She did very well after an initial adjustment. She had several familiar caregivers that came during the day, so she'd have companionship. Even though she was more limited in her conversation, her attitude was good and mostly upbeat, and she maintained her sense of humor. As she declined, she began to speak less and less: using fewer words. She needed lots of help with hygiene and eating. She had a very good medical team and her moods were controlled with a limited amount of medication. Her caregiving team had been with her for the long haul and this gave her comfort.

I don't like to beg, but I am begging you to do one crucial thing for yourself—get help! If you've chosen to care for your family member yourself, find a qualified respite caregiver at the very least. By enlisting the help of others to help during the most difficult times of the disease, you give yourself the gift of presence. You can only be present if you aren't exhausted or overwhelmed all the time. With presence, you will still have many joyful times and beautiful memories with your loved one during this phase. To prevent your own suffering, and the prolonged suffering of your loved one, it will be good to start letting go.

THINGS TO LOOK FOR

Repeating themselves

Losing language

Incontinence

Confabulation, Delusions

WAYS TO PREPARE

FIND A GREAT DOCTOR: Find a neurologist who specializes in dementia or Alzheimer's. This will prevent the situation where your doctor hands you a diagnosis and sends you home to deal with it. A great neurologist will be able to prescribe the right combination of medications to keep your loved one comfortable and enjoying life for as long as possible. If they're comfortable and enjoying life, you will enjoy life more, too. Your local chapter of the Alzheimer's Association may be helpful in making a selection.

In my experience, a good psychiatrist is even more critical to your loved one's comfort, and your sanity, than a neurologist. The psychiatrist will find medication that will help with the behaviors caused by the dementia. I had a client who was very edgy and always ready to be angry. Her psychiatrist prescribed just the right combination of medication that worked very well for her.

Medication

Here is a little talk about medication. It's by no means exhaustive but is a start to the common medications prescribed for dementia and memory loss. There are many combinations of medications that ease the pain of the confusion in both dementia and Alzheimer's disease. Your doctors will prescribe the best ones for your loved one. The most common are cholinesterase inhibitors and memantine.

Cholinesterase Inhibitors improve communications between brain cells and slow memory loss symptoms.

Donepezil (Aricept) is approved for all stages of Alzheimer's.

Rivastigmine (Exelon) is approved to treat mild to moderate Alzheimer's.

Galantamine (Razadyne) is approved to treat mild to moderate Alzheimer's.

Memantine blocks the action of glutamate, a natural substance in the brain that is believed to be linked to symptoms of Alzheimer's disease. Namenda is the brand name for memantine.

There is a now a combination drug called Namzaric. It's a combination of Donepezil and Namenda. Your doctor may prescribe this since it is one pill instead of two. As a combination medication, the dosage is set. If your loved one needs more or less of one of either Donepezil and Namenda, it may not be the best choice.

Antipsychotic medications

There are all kinds of medications for behaviors associated with dementia and Alzheimer's. This may be a trial and error process and not a very fun one.

Symptoms may include uncooperativeness, aggression, agitation, insomnia, hostility to hallucinations and delusions. The person in your care may never have any of these symptoms but it's good to have an overview. There are doctors who are great at finding just the right cocktail for your loved one's situation. Here are a few by name:

aripiprazole(Abilify)

clozapine (Clozaril)

haloperidol (Haldol)

olanzapine (Zyprexa)

quetiapine (Seroquel)

risperidone (Risperdal)

ziprasidone (Geodon)

Urinary Tract Infections

If you see a quick onset of aggression or extreme confusion (delirium), have your loved one checked for a urinary tract infection. Older adults respond differently to a UTI than younger ones. It is thought that typical physical symptoms associated with a UTI are not present with older adults. Instead of painful or more frequent urination or lower back pain, an older adult responds to infection with increased confusion, aggression or withdrawal.

Now that we've covered some key ways to prepare yourself for your loved one's Alzheimer's, you're ready to take on some new communication skills. I promise they will change negative behavior, if you're experiencing it with your loved one, and hopefully, prevent it from happening at all. It's simple, but it might go against your instinctive responses. I hear conversations all over assisted living facilities or with other caregivers and I think to myself, "If only they applied the New Reality Rules!" Well, you get the inside scoop, right here, on how to survive dementia without losing your mind.

CHAPTER 5

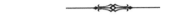

The New Reality Rules

E very day, serving a person with dementia or Alzheimer's as a caregiver, your intention is to maintain and build their self-esteem, reduce fear and anxiety, generate trust and safety, and demonstrate extraordinary kindness. Your job is to know your client well and build communication based on who they are, their values and interests… and to have fun in the process! Always remember that their reality is reality. Explaining why their reality is untrue or wrong will only cause frustration and anger.

You're going to start communicating in a different way with your loved one than you have been. You're going to implement the New Reality Rules.

Dementia has been likened to "having a sliver of your brain sliced off every day." It is painful and terrifying. There is a saying in the dementia world: If a person with dementia is giving you a hard time, it's because they are having a hard time. Remembering this will help you have empathy when they are resisting you, arguing, or getting mad. If they say "I don't want to" it might mean they're afraid or that they have forgotten how to do it.

RULE 1: EMPATHIZE AND VALIDATE THEIR EMOTIONS

The first New Reality Rule is to *Empathize and Validate Their Emotions*. Your job is to speak to the emotion they might be feeling, not react to what they are saying. You're going to use inclusive language to show them that you are in it together and that they are not alone. You're going to put yourself in their shoes.

Your loved one may experience struggles or sadness at times of transitions in care or when you leave. Remembering that people with dementia have greater fears about being left or forgotten (after all, they are forgetting themselves) will help you to empathize with the feeling, rather than reacting to what they say. It may go like this:

Mom: Oh, you're leaving now?

Daughter: Well, I wish I could stay all day, but (caregiver) is here and it would be selfish of me to keep you all to myself! You're going to (go for a walk, do a favorite activity) and then I'm going to be right back! I love you so much! I miss you when I'm not here.

Can you see how this is better than reminding them that you've been with them for hours, days or even if you are their full-time caregiver?

Rather than saying, "I have to go, Mom. I have things to do." Or "I've been here for 10 hours. I need to leave at some point." By addressing the feeling they might be having and expressing your own love and devotion, you speak to their heart and they hear that you love them and that you're coming back.

Empathizing with their emotions will give you more patience and create safety for your loved one. Remembering that their reality is different than yours will help you to step back and feel compassion for what they're feeling.

Using inclusive language, like we and us and not you and your, is another way to empathize with their emotions and fears of being left alone to suffer with their confusion all by themselves. Anything you can do to ease that fear, help them feel secure, and reassure them that they won't be left behind will help.

I had a client who preferred calling her apartment "our place." She felt safer and calmer with that language. So, we always used inclusive language with her, such as, "We need to go to the dentist" and "We're low on yogurt."

RULE 2: MAKE THEM RIGHT

If you haven't already, you will soon learn about the world of endless questions—in a loop. This can be very challenging for a caregiver and can lead to frustration and impatience. Once there's an impatient caregiver, everyone begins to suffer.

When you feel yourself getting impatient, take a breath and count to three. Refrain from answering yes or no to any of the questions and act as if you don't know the answer. Now you're on a journey together to find out the answer. On the journey, you will implement the second New Reality Rule: *Make Them Right*. You're going to provide questions for which your loved one can be right and can answer: Yes!

Here's an example:

Daughter: What did you do today?
Loved One: (looks at caregiver)

Caregiver:	Hmm… What did we do? (Look at and lightly pat the folded laundry on the table)
Loved One:	We did some laundry and folded it!
Caregiver:	We had a lot of laundry, didn't we? What else did we do… hmmm? Did we go to the pharmacy?
Loved One:	Yes! And we saw Tricia at the pharmacy and we gave her a card.
Caregiver:	Yes, we sure did.

This technique puts your loved one in the empowered position of talking about their day instead of having to listen to someone talk for them. It relieves anxiety and frustration and builds their self-esteem. They will like you more, too, because you are "making them right" and this helps them maintain their dignity and self-respect.

RULE 3: LEARN HOW TO LIE

The third New Reality Rule is *Learn How to Lie*. This kind of lying makes all the difference in dealing with people with dementia or Alzheimer's. It is a means of communicating that is deeply empathetic and compassionate. You will definitely not lose your mind if you can learn how to do this right.

Take Josie, for example. Josie loves her caregiver. She is her best friend. She is her memory bank. When her caregiver is around, all is well in the world. When the caregiver leaves, she is anxious. She is terrified and she's mad because she wants things to go her way, always (remember, it's like caring for a toddler and the toddler is in charge. Josie is just like a toddler). At the end of the day, her caregiver has learned some simple ways to make the transition easier. Her reality is that if her caregiver leaves, she will be abandoned.

Caregiver #2 arrives

Caregiver #1: I'm going to take out the trash.

Caregiver #2 gets involved with Josie (conversation or activity)

Caregiver #1 leaves

No goodbye, no fanfare.

Josie is involved in the moment and with Caregiver #2.

This eliminates that moment of fear or feeling of abandonment that Josie feels when someone leaves. It is a kindness to not be honest and straightforward. It is a kindness to lie.

We implemented the same technique on the weekends. Caregiver #1 didn't work on the weekends. So, we lied to show extraordinary kindness and help Josie to feel secure.

Josie: Is (Caregiver #1) coming back?

Caregiver #2: She's definitely coming back! She's coming back bright and early! She misses you too much when she's not here. Why don't we go for our walk now?

Josie had the momentary comfort she was looking for, that caregiver #1 was coming back and in hearing that, Josie could relax. Then they went about the day's activities.

This quick overview of The New Reality Rules gives you an idea of the methods used to ease confusion, anxiety and reduce the fears felt by people with dementia. We'll take a deeper dive into each rule in the next three chapters.

CHAPTER 6

Empathize and Validate Their Emotions

When a person with dementia interacts with another person, their words can sting. We have no idea what we did to deserve what is being dished out. But we also don't know how it would feel to have our brain function decline on a daily basis. how would it feel to be on your way to the bathroom and actually forget that you have to go? To start a sentence, get four words in, and forget your thought? Imagine how frustrating and depressing that would be. Welcome to the mind of a person with dementia.

Compassion, for ourselves and them, and curiosity are required. Looking for what is not being said, the emotions being expressed when the words stab is equally as important. Most negative responses are a result of fear. By looking underneath what's said and looking for the emotion they are feeling, you can communicate with them so they feel safe and secure. Responding to the emotion rather than the words will help you and your loved one and will decrease resistance or anger.

YOU LEFT ME!

I took Claire to the gas station. And I knew it was a risk because Claire hates the gas station. But I was honestly afraid I'd run out of gas and that would be worse. Gas stations are dangerous because of close proximity to strangers and the smell of gas could be a trigger for her. It wasn't crowded so I pulled in and quickly filled up. To keep her occupied, I kept the door open the entire time and we talked about what we'd do next. I got back in the car, thinking, "Whew! We got through that without an upset."

As we pulled away from the station, Claire, started crying, "Why did you leave me? I was scared! I was all alone!! Never leave me like that again!"

I had no idea what she was talking about. I couldn't figure out why she thought I had left her. I had the urge to reason with her and say "I was with you the entire time. We chatted about going to get groceries and going for a walk. What are you talking about?" But I knew that she felt I had left her. She believed what she said. That was her reality. And, I knew she was really sad and scared, so I empathized with her and said, "I am so sorry Claire! I will never leave you again. I want you to feel safe at all times. I'm so sorry you felt unsafe." This stopped her in her tracks. She looked at me in disbelief and said, "That's ok. I'm glad it happened. Now we know what to do next time." Within a few minutes we were singing and laughing again.

At the end of the day, I thought about this incident. The only thing I could come up with was that when her feelings weren't honored, as in her aversion for gas stations, she felt left and disregarded and that feeling of being ignored translated to the feeling of abandonment.

SOMETHING WARM!

Jessie and I were working on a puzzle. It was so impressive to see her focused, turning the pieces, and there was a real feeling of satisfaction when she "click" snapped the pieces into the right spots on the board. It wasn't always easy for her though. Sometimes the puzzle would become too difficult or the pieces wouldn't fall together. Other times she got bored with the activity that would elicit the following Jessie-ism, "Ahhh!

Let's get out of here. Let's get something warm." In Jessie's world, something warm meant food, and not necessarily warm food either. It could mean ice cream, pasta, or something else less than healthy for her, especially if she had just eaten. Now, I knew when we had last eaten and what was consumed. If I went along with her desire for "something warm" every time she said it, she would have had hypertension and weight gain to deal with on top of her Alzheimer's. I had to learn to read between the lines.

When Jessie said she wanted something warm, was she really hungry for food? From observing her, "something warm" was usually preceded by boredom or frustration. Jessie wanted to feel energized, enthusiastic and invigorated!

What worked for me was to pause and then suggest another activity.

Jessie: Let's get something warm.

Me: (Count to three, say NOTHING) Hey, you want to go for a walk? Get some fresh air?

Jessie: That sounds nice.

Suggesting an activity that she likes always worked. I also would make sure we found an activity where she could be validated and excel! So we would head out of her apartment, go for a walk, feed the fish or look at the roses. She could always pick out a rose that smelled good. By the time we were on our way to the rose garden, she had forgotten about "something warm."

I DON'T WANT TO!

Alice was physically able, but her memory loss was completely depressing to her. She could see herself changing, forgetting more and being less able to be involved in her former activities. We talked about volunteering and being of service. She was interested. She honestly wanted to participate but had a hard time committing to anything in the moment that required a schedule.

I committed us to a day for delivering food for the elderly.

I showed up. I told her that today was the day! (mistake)

Then the resistance set in. Her foot hurt, she was hot, she was cold, her wrist hurt. Her pants were too tight. Her pants were too loose.

She was doing everything she could do to not show up.

As you can imagine it was very difficult for me. My mind was racing with all kinds of frustrations and recriminations and wanting to cancel. I had planned on having plenty of extra time to get ready, knowing she might be resistant. I knew it would be good for her, so I literally breathed through all of her resistance and got her out the hardest door to get through: our own. I knew that once we started, she would be a different person. We arrived, gathered our lunches and drove to meet five seniors in our community.

Alice was smitten. She just loved each and every one of our recipients and felt so accomplished by being of service.

It might be that your loved one doesn't want to see family they haven't seen in a while. I've heard from many clients, whether their loved ones have dementia or Alzheimer's, that they're afraid because they know they can't keep up with a conversation or that they might not know what to do in a new activity or environment. Or that someone might find out that they aren't remembering. Reassure them with words like, "We'll be together the whole time. We'll just go for a little while and then we can leave when we want to." Knowing that you're on their side and will stand by them can comfort them and ease their fear. Once they're in the moment, they will probably be fine. Be prepared to make a quick getaway if necessary.

We've covered some scenarios for New Reality Rule 1: Validate and Empathize with their Emotions. Now we'll delve into Rule #2: Make Them Right.

CHAPTER 7

Make Them Right

Not having to be right has saved me from many arguments with clients, and also led to more peace and joy in the relationships. Being right makes the other person wrong, right? How would you feel if someone who made you feel wrong showed up day after day? My guess is you wouldn't like it, and you wouldn't like the person who made you feel that way. Possibly just seeing them walk through the door would put you on edge and make you angry. You probably really wouldn't want to see them, truth be told. If you don't process words and feelings in a typical way, it might make you furious.

Let's face it, we don't like know-it-alls. I was guilty of being a know-it-all with one of my clients. It was all with good intentions. I wanted to be helpful, but I was actually humiliating and infuriating. Thankfully, I learned a better way.

I learned that I don't have to be right. This technique can be a lot of fun if you let it. Take a journey with your loved one to find out the answers to questions. It brings you closer to one another and helps you both experience peace and joy.

YOU'VE GOT MAIL!

Lara loved to get messages from friends and family. She would check her phone repeatedly for updates and often asked to go to the post office to check the mail.

One day, we received a text from Lara's sister. They went back and forth several times with a little assistance from me. Lara was just thrilled to hear from her sister and smiled about it for most of the day. When it came time for the shift change, the next caregiver wanted to know how the day went. We told her about all we did and then I mentioned the messages from Lara's sister.

"I didn't hear from my sister," she said sternly.

"Oh, (smiling)...yes. We did! It's still in your phone."

I brought the phone over, still not recognizing her frustration. We scrolled through the messages and found the thread with her sister on it.

"See?" I said cheerfully. "We found out that she has been taking care of her neighbor's dog."

Lara interrupted me. "I didn't see those. We didn't talk to her. You should leave now. You aren't helping me right now. I have a headache. I'm going to lay down."

I felt horrible. I had obviously upset her and I was only trying to help.

I sat in my car and cried. I called the Alzheimer's Association for help and I will never forget what the amazing social worker told me when I relayed the story to her. As she explained to me what might have been going on for Lara, I realized what I had done.

From Lara's viewpoint, I knew something she didn't know and that was annoying and frustrating to her. It reminded her that she didn't remember. Not only did I know something she didn't know, I showed her in black and white that she had forgotten. This was so upsetting for her that she sent me packing and had to lay down to relieve her stress. Knowing more than your loved ones or clients know reminds them that they don't remember. It dishonors them and makes them feel stupid.

What I learned, is to never remind. Be right where they are. This is how those conversations go now.

Friend: How was your day? What happened?

Caregiver: **(Count to 3 SAY NOTHING.** Give your loved one the chance to say whatever they want to say)

Your loved one looks at you

Caregiver: Hmmmmmm…what did we do today? Did we go for a walk?

Client: Oh Yes! We went for a walk today. We saw a bluebird.

Caregiver: That's right! Wasn't that beautiful?

If there is more. Start again.

Caregiver: Hmmmm…what else happened? Did we talk with anyone? Jane? Did we talk with Jane?

Client: I don't think so. I wonder how she's doing?

Caregiver: Let's send her a message tomorrow and say hi.

Now we're in it together. It isn't me remembering and Lara not remembering. It's us working together to remember what happened. It's Lara being honored and acknowledged and included in the recounting of the day's activities.

Does it really matter that Lara had heard from her sister? Not really.

At some point, she will go through her messages, see the texts and then get excited all over again when she realizes it for herself. So letting her be "right" and not arguing or knowing more than she does gives her an even greater sense of joy and control.

LET'S GET PAPER TOWELS!

Barbara, mentioned earlier in this book, was an Amazon Addict! She loved to shop and she loved using Amazon. We were always fully stocked with paper towels, toilet paper and any household items we could possibly use. For some reason paper towels were a favorite product.

Barbara: I think we need paper towels.

Me: **(Count to 3)** Hmmmm…ok. We might need some other things, too. Let's have a look.

We walk through the house together.

Me: Oh, (opens overflowing cabinets) here are the paper towels.

Barbara: Oh, wow! We have plenty. What about toothpaste?

In this step, remember: you don't know more than they do...ever. Anything they see for the first time, even if you've both seen it 2,019 times, is being seen for the first time together.

LET'S EAT!

The story mentioned in the last chapter about Jessie also applies to this rule. When Jessie forgets that she's eaten, she will forage through the refrigerator, take everything out and snack a little. When we clean up and put everything away, she says, "I wonder what there is to eat? What do we have in here?"

Jessie isn't hungry...we know this. What do we say? Do we let her eat and eat, hoping that she will feel full? Here's what has worked best for us:

Jessie: When are we going to eat? Let's get some food.

Me: **(Count to 3)** Hmmmmm...ok, we'll eat soon. Can you help me fold this laundry?

It is our natural tendency to correct someone who says something that doesn't make sense in our reality. It isn't "true," so we want to correct it and be right. The reason this doesn't work is that Jessie doesn't remember that she just ate. She doesn't remember. If I said, "We just ate," she would be embarrassed and angry and she probably wouldn't believe me. She might get mad or she might just think that I never feed her.

It is better to redirect the activities and tell her we *will* eat. Now her feelings and statement have been honored, and since she isn't actually hungry, we can get on with another activity until it is time to eat.

Here's another...

IN THE RESTROOM

Your loved one uses the toilet. You're a perceptive caregiver and are listening. You didn't hear the faucet run, so you know that hands weren't washed. You could say, "Don't forget to wash your hands," and now you have reminded them that they forgot and they are mad at you.

Instead, try saying, "Wow, I really need to wash my hands!"

Turn on the water, "Oh, it's nice and warm and this soap smells so good. Try some!"

This next one is my favorite...

IS THIS MY HOUSE?

My grandfather had Alzheimer's. This was over 30 years ago, and once he couldn't live at home anymore, he lived in a hospital setting. It was awful. My mom visited him often and I sometimes went along. I couldn't go often because it was too painful for me to see him like that. He lived in a completely different reality and it was difficult for me to watch at the time. Now when I think about it, it was actually a blessing that he believed he was in his home back in New York.

Similarly, I met a woman through the academy who lived with her mother and experienced the same type of confusion as my grandpa. Her daughter was exhausted and hadn't had any training. Here are how the conversations went before she learned a better way.

Mom: (confused) Is this my house?

Daughter: Yes, Mom this is your house.

Mom: (confused and distressed) Do I live here?

Daughter: Yes, Mom you live here. I live here with you.

Mom: Are my parents here?

Daughter: No, Mom. Your parents have been dead for a long time.

Mom: (sad and frustrated) Oh. When I get up in the morning, will I know that this is my house?

Daughter: No, I'll wake you up in the morning and tell you that this is your house.

Mom: Oh. (turns and walks away, muttering.)

Here's how the conversation goes when you're *Making Them Right*.

Mom: Is this my house?

Daughter: Hmmm…I've been wondering that too. Let's look around and see where we are.

(Daughter leads mom to a photo of her mom with her favorite grandchild, pet, painting from her room, etc.) Hmmm… have you seen this? What is this?

Mom: That's Scottie! My dog.

Daughter: Yes! Scottie was a good dog.

Mom: Yes, he was.

Daughter: Hmmmm…was that picture taken at your house?

Mom: Yes! It was in the backyard.

Daughter: Yes, it was taken right by that tree (pointing out the window) in your backyard.

Mom: That's right. This is my backyard.

Daughter: Yes, it sure is. Hey! Look at this? Is this your chair?

Mom: Yes, my favorite chair.

Daughter: Why don't you sit down in your favorite chair and I'll make us some tea.

Now you're off in a different direction—a positive one—where your loved one feels validated and you have done that just by how you talk to her.

What is the difference here? Notice how many "yes" answers are in the second conversation. Notice who is answering the questions. It's the mom, not her daughter. This is a much more empowering way to speak to a person with dementia. Does this mean that you will go through it fewer times? No. Your loved one is still going to forget. But what they won't forget is that they feel good when they talk to you. They aren't being told that they are wrong all the time. How many people like to be told "no" all the time?

Contradicting a person's beliefs or reality is insanity and creates a very unhappy client and one who might lash out or become withdrawn. Nobody can really say, but we can try to put ourselves in their position. Imagine you thought the sky was green and you were with someone who, every time you said, "Isn't that a beautiful green sky?" said to you "That's blue, not green." A few minutes later you said, "I just love this green sky today." Then they say again, "I just told you that's blue. That's a blue sky." It would be obvious that you just can't agree and since they are the ones correcting you, you must be wrong.

The key is to use communication as a means to empower them and that helps them to figure out the answers. Your language and behavior can either support them or it can tear them down.

You get to make the choice.

CHAPTER 8

Learn How to Lie

I am an honest person. I value straightforward, honest communication. I was taught to always tell the truth and to never lie! I was taught that lying is bad and even sinful. Parents and children, spouses who have lived together for decades, and compassionate caregivers can't imagine not being truthful with each other.

Most of us have an innate sense that we need to be truthful. The idea of lying, especially to someone we love, is repugnant to us. There is a morality that we all have about lying to our loved ones. It's a good thing to have, but when our loved ones have dementia, lying, when used appropriately, becomes our ally in helping them feel secure and safe.

Although I value honesty, I also value kindness and empathy. In dealing with people with dementia, balancing our beliefs about honesty and our role in contributing to their feeling safe can be a slippery slope to walk. Sometimes the kindest thing to do is to tell a lie. The kind of lying I'm talking about here is not a destructive lie, but an expression of extraordinary kindness. The examples that follow will clarify New Reality Rule #3: Learn How To Lie.

DON'T GO!

Many caregivers deal with difficult transition times when leaving their client or loved one. I met a client through the academy that had miraculous success using this technique. His wife had been moved into memory care in the assisted living facility where they were living together. He spent a great amount of time with her every day. Goodbye time was very stressful for both of them.

Jack and Ginny were a very devoted couple. They were still adjusting to not living together. They had a routine of walking, having breakfast, watching a program and then Ginny's caregiver came to relieve Jack for a few hours. When he got up to leave, his wife would panic and snap, "Where are you going? Why are you leaving? When are you coming back?"

His honest response, "I'm going back to my room and then I'm going out for a while and then I'll be back."

"You're going where? What do you mean 'your room?' You're leaving me here? I'm going with you."

"Dear, I'll be back before you know it. You won't even know I'm gone."

"Just leave. You are selfish. Just go!"

They had always been honest with one another. He didn't know any other way to be than honest. He was distraught. He didn't know how to answer her. He didn't want to upset her, but he didn't know what do.

He learned how to lie.

This was very difficult for him. He longed to have his wife back, the one who could understand coming and going. But as he experienced her panic, he saw that the only way to change the outcome was to change himself. He wanted her to experience peace and calm. He wanted to express as much kindness as he could. He decided that she needed to hear something other than what he considered the truth.

His wife is afraid. Her reality has shifted. She is afraid of being left behind and forgotten. She has all kinds of other fears we aren't aware of and don't experience because our brains are not being slowly shaved away. When we must leave, a "lie" gives them instantaneous comfort in that moment because in the next moment they are occupied with what is in front of them. They need to feel and believe that you are not leaving them. Each moment is the moment they are in. So, if each moment is peaceful and calm, then their lives are peaceful and calm.

THE NEW WAY:

Jack: I'm going to take out the trash. I'll be right back.

Ginny looks up, then goes back to her activity.

Jack leaves.

Ginny is cheerfully engaged with her caregiver. He does errands and takes some respite time. He returns three hours later.

Ginny: (Smiling) Have you seen (TV program)?

Jack: I haven't! (He has, but he *Makes Her Right*)

He sits, and they watch TV together.

Another way of transitioning is to have the next caregiver become quickly engaged with your loved one and then for you to leave quietly without even saying goodbye. If your loved one is distracted with something they enjoy, they don't really know that you have gone. If they ask later, the caregiver can say,

"Oh, he just stepped out and will be back soon to (go for a walk, watch XYZ) with you. Can you help me (favorite activity, fold laundry, wash dishes)? How about we make some tea? Would you like Earl Grey or cinnamon apple?"

It also works if you or the primary caregiver will be gone for an extended amount of time or if your loved one has weekend caregivers. On Friday it's best to say, "See you bright and early tomorrow!" even if you won't see them bright and early.

Your loved one wants in-the-moment reassurance that they aren't being left or forgotten. As long as they believe in the moment that you're coming back, all is well. By the time they realize you are gone, they aren't upset because they didn't have to feel the feeling of being left. When you come back, it's as if no time has passed.

I WANT TO SEE MY MAMA

Your loved ones may have forgotten that their parents are dead. They may ask to go see them. Now, we have a choice to make and the first thing to remember is your explaining the "truth" to them is not going to change their reality. If you tell the truth, "Mom, your mother has been dead for 40 years," you run the risk of making them feel stupid and people don't like people who make them feel stupid. Another thing to consider is that for a person with dementia, a reminder of a painful event that happened yesterday or 20 years ago is processed as if it is happening right now. What does that mean? If they are told about their parents' death, they will experience the grief and loss as if it is happening at that very moment. Then they will forget…and ask again. Now you're in a vortex of upset, grief and sadness.

The solution:

Mom: I want to see my mama. Let's go for a visit.

Daughter: You're missing your mama? (*Empathizing with Emotions*)

Mom: Yes, and she makes the best apple pie.

Daughter: She does make the best apple pie. Let's go see her tomorrow. Today, we need to get some things done around here.

Mom: Ok.

OR:

Mom: I want to see my mama. Let's go for a visit.

Daughter: Your parents are wonderful people, I'd like to see them, too. Let's figure out a time to visit while we have some tea?

THE FARMERS' MARKET

I had a client who obsessed over farmers' markets. If we let her, she would go to a farmers' market every day. She loved the fresh food and the crowd and excitement of it all. Living in Santa Barbara, she could actually go to a farmer's market every day if she wanted to!

So, we had to *Learn How to Lie* about it.

Jane: Is there a farmers' market today?

Me: Hmmmm… we have a farmers' market the day after tomorrow. Let's look at what we have here. (Open refrigerator) We have berries, figs, oranges and avocados.

Jane: Oh wow! We're loaded!

10 minutes later…

Jane: Do we have a farmers' market today?

Lather. Rinse. Repeat.

Now you've prevented an upset. How?

You haven't contradicted your loved one. Your lying to them has them feel validated and then they can make the momentary decision that is appropriate. You haven't given them a reason to fight with you.

Your loved ones will feel taken care of when we tell them we'll be right back. We help them when we prevent them from doing things that aren't in their best interest. We show love when we live in their reality.

It is worth overcoming our resistance to lying because this kind of lying is an act of kindness. It requires a deep knowing of your client or loved one, which we already have or are developing. Once we know their triggers and their safe words, we can work to create more peace, calm and joy in our newly changed relationships with them. When they have peace and calm, so do their caregivers.

CHAPTER 9

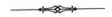

For Caregivers Only

"The best way to find yourself is to lose yourself in the service of others."

—Mahatma Gandhi

"Being of service to others is what brings true happiness."

—Marie Osmond

"When you're in the service of your fellow beings, you're in the service of God."

—Anonymous

I f you have been called as a caregiver and you have answered that call, you are on a blessed journey of service. There is nothing like knowing the difference you are making in the life of an individual with dementia and the contribution you are to the family of that loved one. You have a great purpose on your new journey. You are the memory bank and connection to the world for a person with dementia. As they slip away, day by day, you are there as a safety net. It is an important role to play in the life of another. Embrace it and give it the weight it deserves. Every day, as a caregiver, your goal is to build self-esteem, reduce fear and anxiety, and generate trust and safety. Your job is to know your client well, to build friendship and trust, and develop communication based on who they are, their values and interests. Your job is also to have fun!

THE CARE AND KEEPING OF YOU

First of all, you must manage your own self-care. You cannot be of service to others if you aren't taking care of yourself. Are you getting the appropriate exercise, eating healthy foods, staying hydrated, and taking breaks for renewal? Most caregivers are so busy being and doing for others that they neglect these fundamental elements of care. We all know the old adage "Put your own mask on first." If you don't take care of you, there will be nothing left for you to give to someone else. There are plenty of ways to do self-care.

It might involve getting up a few minutes earlier each day. Please value yourself enough to do this.

When I first started the work of caregiving, I felt that I was disappearing…and I was. Caring for a person with dementia is all about them, and that is appropriate. They are totally reliant on you and can be self-absorbed and self-centered. It really is like caring for a two-year-old and the two-year-old is in charge. There is a phenomenon that's akin to melding together. They see you as an extension of themselves. In their mind, you don't exist apart from them and vice versa.

Take Breaks

A friend of mine who lives with her father finds respite in her job. Ultimately, you'll want to get help so that you can take a break and do something that refreshes you. If you are working privately, you'll need to have very good boundaries so that you don't become overworked. If you are a trustworthy, reliable caregiver, you have no idea the contribution you are to the family you serve. They will want you seven days a week, 24 hours a day! Learn how to graciously say no and offer other options for them when you can't be there. Build a network of other reliable, trustworthy caregivers so you can help each other.

Please find a venting and brainstorming buddy or a support group where you can be heard, talk about the struggles you are having and know that you are not alone. When you find a support group, make sure it's one where good ideas are shared and not one where people only share the horror stories. You don't want to be taking care of the people in your support group, too! You need to find hope and support.

What are the ways you like to give yourself care? Do those things! Meditate, rest, exercise and eat well. Be as good a caregiver to yourself as you are to others.

KEEP THEM MOVING!

Do your best to keep your client active and engaged in the world. What are their favorite activities? Music can be a great way to connect and stimulate memory. I have had many two-person dance parties over the years! Playing music from when they were young or any music that makes you smile will promote good vibes and good feelings. These shared positive experiences will carry you through during the tough times. Taking walks is good for body and soul. Enjoying the fresh air, sights and sounds and greeting people going by does so much for you and for your client. It gets you moving and your endorphins flowing.

If the person you are caring for played sports or enjoyed a particular physical activity (golf, bowling, dance, walking, shuffleboard, etc.), is there a way they can still be involved? Can the activity be modified so they can still participate? Muscle memory is strong. The release of endorphins during and after physical activity will raise their mood as well as give them a great sense of satisfaction by engaging in a familiar physical activity. I saw it with one of my clients who was an amazing athlete. Kerry, mentioned in the introduction, had won tournaments in her younger years and when she got on the court, it all came back to her. She was in complete flow. Her self-esteem and energy was off the charts after playing. It was a beautiful thing to see.

Your loved ones may resist, but using the systems in Chapters 5-8 really work to overcome their resistance to activities that are good for them. Keeping the results in mind, recognizing the value in the activity and what they'll get from it, and also acknowledging the frustration you may feel, will help you to deal with the resistance.

Going for drives has been another way to keep the mind engaged and can be a relaxing activity when anxiety sets in. Drive slowly. If possible, pick streets or areas that are scenic. My Mom and other clients love to read the street signs. If you're driving through familiar areas, they will tell you the stories connected with the places en route. It also gives you a little break.

GET RELATED!

In getting to know your client, you want to know more than the medical aspects of their care.

Who are they as people? What are their interests? How have they contributed to the world in their lives? What are their stories? What are their values? Getting to know your client, so that they become your loved one, is a joyful journey.

Tess, mentioned earlier in this book, was my very first client. We spent a few hours together every day. Each week I spoke to her daughter to let her know how things were going. As I was recounting our activities, I told her, "Your mom told me all about growing up in the Central Valley, and that they had two mini Schnauzer's, but they weren't allowed in the house." I went on and on with details about her stories. Ann told me, in surprise, "My mom never talked about that! I never knew that she had dogs growing up."

You have a precious role as a person's caregiver and companion. They will share things with you that they don't share with others. I suggest you keep a small journal to capture the gems you will learn about them as they share stories of their life.

Being with a person who is changing and losing parts of themselves, it's especially important to develop the language that they begin to use. This is another intimate part of the role you play as caregiver. Knowing what they mean and are trying to communicate as they begin to lose language is vital. Use the words that they use. It becomes a secret language that you share and creates a beautiful bond between you.

CARING VS. OVER-CARING

Most people who are caregivers are caregivers because they are caregivers. They have a natural inclination to help and to serve. While the intention comes from love, it can unintentionally do damage to your client.

I was holding a regular staff meeting, and one of my caregivers told me,

"When I order food for Angie, I look straight at the server and say, "When you bring the food, put it all in front of me. Don't put it in front of her. I ask them for a cup of ice. When the food comes, I put some ice in the soup and stir it up. I cool it off and then I give it to Angie. I tell her, 'It's cool now, you can eat it.' Then I take her food, I cut it up nice and small and hand it to her so she can eat it."

I nearly lost my #$%& and punched a hole through the wall! I honestly was completely floored and stunned. This is not my model. Let me explain.

Angie has Alzheimer's and she is a very capable adult woman. She's social, participates in many activities, is very bright and she certainly knows (at least for now) how to behave in a dining room, cut her own food and eat.

I believe and demand that my caregivers treat an adult as an adult. As people with dementia change, their habits and preferences change. Sometimes they pick outfits that I wouldn't pick. Maybe they want to wear a heavy coat in the summer. Pick your battles. They are adults who have the right to exercise their choices as long as it isn't hurting themselves or anyone else.

Angie's other caregivers give her the space to be herself. We use "I Don't Have to Be Right" when in the dining room together and guess what? Angie doesn't need her $%^#$ food cut up! She is perfectly capable of eating by herself. There may come a day when she can't, but until then, we honor her by allowing her to have independence and do what she can for herself.

Even with the best of intentions, a caregiver's "over-caring" creates less independence for the person receiving care. It takes away opportunity for them to do the things they still can do and to experience the dignity and self-esteem for doing things for themselves.

Don't assume that you know what your client wants. A person with dementia is still a person. By observing first and stepping back, a caregiver, whether it's a family member or someone hired, can really assess what needs to be done. To provide respectful care, the caregiver really needs to slow down and observe. It may seem easier or quicker to do it yourself, but this really isn't in your loved one's best interest.

TIPS OF THE TRADE

The Angry Client: Play Hide and Seek

No matter what you do, there will be times when your client will get angry. It's part of the disease. I had a very challenging client who got mad and would slam doors, yelling and muttering. She was safe and not in harm's way, so I waited in a different room quietly. After a few minutes, she came out and said, "Anyone here?" I'd say, "Here I am," not really knowing what the response would be. Nine times out of ten, she'd say, "Hi! When did you get here?" She completely forgot what she was mad about and was ready to move on with her day. On that 10th time when she came out mad, I'd repeat the process and soon she would be cheerful again.

Showers

Caregivers of people with dementia or Alzheimer's at some point will talk about their loved one not wanting to take a shower. I haven't met one who hasn't had this challenge. There are many theories about why. Some say it's because they can't see the water, and it's scary to have an invisible force hitting their skin. Some say that the process of getting into the shower is upsetting because they feel cold or exposed. I had a client refuse a shower for many days. When she finally got in, she didn't know what to do. She had forgotten what to do in the shower.

I say pick your battles. Unless considerable hygiene or health issues arise or you have a family who insists that your client showers on a particular schedule, who cares if someone takes a few days off from a shower? If you're lucky, they will forget that they thought the water was contaminated or whatever their fear is, and eventually get in the shower. There are many tips that people use based on knowing the fears of their particular loved one.

Make sure the room is warm and that the towels are warm. Have them sit in a shower chair. Start with the handheld showerhead at their feet and move upwards. Use dry shampoo and sponge baths in between showers.

You can change your attitude about being in public with someone who looks like they're on the wild side. It is a practice in acceptance. It can be pretty fun to see the looks you get and it makes for a great story later!

Slow Down and Let Them Lead the Way

I have a client who loves to go out and getting ready to go out is sometimes is day-long event! She puts on clothes and then wants to change them because they're too tight or she's cold (in 90-degree weather). Once we get out the door, she may want to change again. We go back inside, making sure we have all of our supplies: tissues, eye drops, breath drops, water, a scarf, sunscreen. After spending quite a bit of time with her and her having outbursts because we didn't have the eye drops she needs ("we should *always* have plenty of eye drops. *Always!*"), I could easily get frustrated or tell her what to wear. But one of the secrets of having the most joy in care giving, and for your loved one, is just to let them be. I actually find it charming to see her change her clothes and be so thoughtful about what she wants to wear. We just take as much time as we need to.

Another client of mine is obsessed with safety. One time I tripped when I was with her and she never forgot it, so when she's outside and sees acorns or olives or palm kernels, she will brush them to the side with her foot or bend down and pick them up. It's pretty amusing to watch because there might be a thousand acorns on the ground and it does not deter her. She will try to pick up all of them and is satisfied when the street is clean with no tripping hazards. I could become impatient or even embarrassed by this seemingly odd behavior. However, I allow her to continue to be herself. As long as she isn't in danger and isn't hurting herself or others, she should be allowed to take her time during her day to do the things she wants to do.

COMMUNICATION AND CONNECTION

I love saying things like, "Sorry, you can't get rid of me! I'm here to stay (with a smile)!"

When another caregiver is coming onto a shift I say, "Well, I'd like to be selfish and stay with you all day and night, but (insert name) wants to spend time with you, too. I'll be back bright and early!" This simple communication has made a world of difference in the relationships built with clients. I want them to hear my words in their ears and minds: that I love being with them, I'm always coming back and that I'm on their side.

WORKING WITH FAMILIES: BE THE BUDDHA

Respect Values and Property

Floored. Completely floored. A woman I met in a support group told me about her dad. He was an ex-military man and fastidious in his home and property. Her mom has Alzheimer's and they had respite care for both of them so that he would not be a full-time caregiver. Each has different skills…and annoying habits. One sing-songs all the time and calls them "sweetie" and "honey" but she's very organized and keeps the household running smoothly. The other one has a calmer disposition but bulldozes dad in decision making and she leaves pen marks on the sofa from doing crossword puzzles!

You are working in someone else's home. Respect the way they do things. Respect their property. If they want all the appliances unplugged every night, then do it. If they want the floor cleaned with Clorox every day, then do it.

What will make you a standout caregiver is regularly asking for feedback on your performance. Accept the feedback, do what your family wants done and do it their way.

Politics and Religion

I wish I didn't have to put this in here, but alas, I do. Don't discuss politics or religion with your client's family, especially if you don't agree. I worked with a caregiver who did this. She was evangelistic about her views and went head-to-head with the family we worked for. She got fired.

Dynamics

Families…we all have them. From our favorite aunt to our weird cousin to our loving (or controlling) mother. We don't get to choose them and that's the same for working with a family.

There might be someone who is a thorn in your side—and guess what? You get to deal with that. That gets to be part of your personal growth. As long as your client is not in danger, your job is to abide by the family's instructions and values. You're going to meet people in their lives who don't know the communication skills you're learning and aren't interested in learning them. Your client will get anxious before, during and after seeing them and it is your job to manage those emotions before, during and after any visits with them. The dynamics between family members started long before you and you won't change them. If you can accept them for what they are, you will be successful.

Remember Kerry from the beginning of this book? She had a person in her life who was completely clueless. When I met him, I was appalled at the way he treated her. He was controlling and disrespectful and I didn't trust him. He talked about her in the third person right in front of her. Here's how it went:

Him (to me): So today, she's going to go to lunch with me, but stay at her place. Then maybe tomorrow you can bring her back over here. And then we'll figure out if she's staying at her place or over here.

As this monologue went on, Kerry got more and more upset and I got more and more concerned about her safety with such a person. After he finished talking, which took a while, I stepped back, looked at Kerry, and basically translated.

Looking at Kerry, I said: Ok, so Joe wants to have lunch with you and then you and I will go back to our place and figure out the rest of the day. Does that sound good to you?

Kerry (still confused): Yes, that's fine.

Kerry was really reticent about seeing him most days (ya think??), but there were times when she did want to see him. For the most part, her family supported the relationship. He was also one of the few people who consistently showed up for her and that was an important role. He had no interest in attending any training or workshops, and made it clear that he wouldn't be a "caregiver" for her. It was very difficult for me. I wanted to support Kerry and had to navigate a very strange dynamic between her and Joe.

I did the only thing I could do.

I was the Buddha and led by example.

When Joe and Kerry and I were together, I modeled the kind of communication that included Kerry. I modeled patience and compassion for Joe even though I really didn't want to. He was losing Kerry just the way the rest of us were and I felt his pain.

It actually made a difference.

Pretty soon, his language changed. I noticed him trying to talk to her the way I did. I think he saw the difference in her anxiety when that kind of communication was used. The (very) small changes he made were encouraging and it made a difference for Kerry.

In dealing with all people, family and friends of your clients, you are the Buddha. You sit in openness and with no judgment. You can listen to all sides but take no side.

Even if family members don't know how to treat their loved one, isn't it better that the relationships stay intact than having no relationship at all? Remember that family is family.

Family dynamics are just that. You won't change any family members. Some may want to learn how to better care for their loved one and some won't. Make peace with all the players: friends, family, significant others, even if they stress your client. They are there and your role is to manage your client in spite of people who mean well.

REMEMBER

People with dementia aren't being hard on you, they are having a hard time.

You can't control a person with dementia. You can only be with them and learn how to manage their complex emotions and behavior. Their experience and behavior are largely dependent on the quality of their care. If your client is anxious and "behaving badly," you will need to change something...and that something is probably you. Get some training in communication or attend a reliable support group. Do *something*.

You are the memory bank and the keeper of the joy and fun. You are everything. You have great responsibility. With you in their life, your client will keep all that they can of their original selves and be allowed to be who they are now.

CHAPTER 10

For Families Only

I got a call from my friend, Beth, late on a Friday afternoon. I was so happy to see her name on the caller ID, but as soon as I picked up, I knew this wouldn't be our typical friendly chat. She was serious, quiet and not herself. She was scared.

"I got a call today from my mom's neighbor. He said he saw my mom in his garden, pulling weeds and shaking her head. He went out and talked to her and she asked him, "Why are those flowers there? I didn't plant them. I don't even like day lilies." He was sort of speechless. Finally, he said, "um..Mrs. Knight, I planted these flowers. This is my yard." My mom flinched and her eyes got big and then she laughed and made a little comment to cover herself and went home. He called me right away and I then called my mom. She seems totally fine now, but I know that we're going to have to see a doctor for some follow-up. I'm scared to death of what I'm going to find out."

I tried to reassure her and give her some comfort without really knowing what was going on, but we both knew that something was up. She made the call to her mom's family doctor and a neurologist. And then she waited.

She called me again a few weeks later. Her bad news got worse.

"She has Alzheimer's," Beth told me. Now her panic streamed out.

"What am I going to do? I am freaking out. I can't quit my job; I have my own kids to raise! What's going to happen to her...to us...to me? Is she going to have to move in? I don't know if I can do that...but she needs me. How much is this all going to cost? Can she even live on her own anymore? She seemed perfectly fine the last time I saw her, but I don't live that close. Did I miss something? Was I too self-absorbed and going along my merry way and all the while there were signs I was missing? How will I handle this and still function in my own life? How much worse will she get? How much time do we have with her?" And on it went and the tears flowed.

Maybe you're like Beth and have just heard some bad news. Or maybe you're anticipating news like this based on signs you're seeing with a parent or loved one. Chances are you're scared, maybe even terrified. You've heard the stories or are living them yourself… stories of wandering, falling, getting lost. At the very least you may have a parent or loved one who is asking the same question over and over, losing independence and becoming more and more childlike.

You're afraid you'll have to make some hard decisions: Can Mom stay in her house? Will she have to move in with family? With you? Into a facility? How will you stay ahead of it? Will your family be there to help or not? How will you keep from resenting the people who stop showing up? How can you continue to live your life and also make sure that your parent or loved one gets what they need?

Planning ahead and taking action will help. If you're seeing signs, get your loved one to a doctor. They may resist you, so you can start using the communication tips in this book to help you. They are afraid, too.

I've met so many families that are struggling to find the right situation for their loved one. What works best for you? Do your parents want to live in their home? Are they ready to move into a place where they will have more help available to them? It really is possible to create a situation where they continue to have independence and thrive, whether it's in their own home or in a new place that will become home.

If your loved one wants to stay home and you're afraid for their safety, there are precautions you can take. It's really sticky with the early stages, and actually, it gets easier once they're further progressed in the disease. When you're dealing with a person who isn't aware of their dementia, or is trying hard to keep it hidden from you, it is very, very difficult. Being available or having friends stop by daily to check in will be your best defense to keeping your family member safe in those earlier stages.

DISABLE THE STOVE

"She can't live in a house or an apartment. What if she turns on the stove and walks away? I can't take on that liability. She has to be in assisted living!"

We hear horror stories of Mom putting on a pot of tea and then forgetting that it's there. Some families decide at this point that it's time to move mom and dad to assisted living, but there are other ways. Get an electric kettle that turns itself off. Have food delivered. There are plenty of services that do this, including free ones for seniors. Prepare mini-meals or snacks in the refrigerator for convenience. Fill a gallon jug of water with a spigot each day with a note: "Drink this until it is empty!"

GET RID OF THE CAR

"I can drive. I'm perfectly capable!"

If your loved one is actually not safe behind the wheel, it might be time to sell it or take the car to another location where he or she can't see it every day. Give them a set of keys that doesn't work and use the New Reality Rules. *Empathize* with their desire for continued independence and allow them all the independence they can have.

If they ask if they will ever drive again, say, "… hmmm? What do you think?" and then change the subject. *Learn How to Lie* and tell your loved one that the car is in the shop and will be back soon. Keep them, and others, safe.

DEMENTIA PROOF THE HOUSE

You won't believe the products available for safety proofing your home. Simple clocks that give time, with AM or PM, day of the week, date. Big button remote controls. Locks for cabinets and doors.

If your loved one is up at night, do all you can to allow them to be safe in their new reality and also let others in the house get the sleep they need. Safety proof the house and let them roam. You can prepare by having limited amounts of food available, so they don't overeat. If they have the big button remote and can use it, they can watch a program. There are technologies available that can give just one or two choices (news and westerns) so that your loved one can choose the program they want to watch on their own.

Stock the table with activities: puzzles, activity boards, coloring supplies, and whatever else keeps their interest. Sometimes even a pile of towels to be folded can be a satisfying activity for your loved one. Keeping their minds and hands engaged in activity, at night or during the day, will make for more peace and calm for all.

The next level of safety-proofing includes alarm enabled floor mats that sound when they're stepped on, motion sensors, monitors and good locks, some with alarms, for the doors.

HAVE FUN!

The other thing to remember is that there is still a lot of fun to be had. There's a lot of joy and life left! The families I've worked with have learned the skills to continue to enjoy their loved ones, even in the changed state that they're in. One wonderful caregiver goes to dance class with her mom each week. They have the best time and giggle and laugh, like old friends. I enjoy many sweet moments with my mom. We paint together (she's a great artist). She guides me and teaches me. It's great for both of us. Another family caregiver is astonished at the closeness she feels with her dad. She relates, "Taking care of him has created this whole new relationship. It's a deeper bond. I really miss my mom, but I know that when my dad goes, it will be much harder because of all the time we've spent together. It's been an amazing journey."

We haven't addressed how you will still live your life. It's up to you to give that to yourself. This is where good help comes in, either in extended family or outside support.

If you're going to care for your loved one yourself, please refer to the chapter for caregivers. Please join a support group and get a little training. Respite support will be invaluable and is an absolute must! Make a schedule and stick to it. You don't want to get overwhelmed or burned out. Get your exercise and nourish yourself physically and spiritually, do the things that bring you respite. I have met so many families that work together beautifully, including extended family and in-laws, in caring for a family member with dementia. One caregiver I met is engaged to be married. She moved out of her home with her partner to live with her father. Her fiancé comes and does shifts so that she can have a break. Her father got the flu and was sick for days. She and her fiancé changed the sheets multiple times during the night, then got up and went to work the next day. I met a caregiver who took care of her mother and is now taking care of her father. She has an amazing family, too. Her children, who are young adults, do shifts with their grandmother, and her in-laws help, too. She works full-time and is a full-time caregiver as well. She has a lot of support, and I admire their family values and her loyalty and strength.

EXPECTATIONS OF OTHER FAMILY MEMBERS

It isn't always like that for families. Many families fall apart because one sibling feels the other or others don't pull their weight. When responsibility lands heavily on one family member, resentments can build. Finding a way to have support so that you aren't overwhelmed can help you have compassion for a family member that simply can't do more than they are doing. I believe that family members really do their best. If there is emotional distance or inability to show up and help, it's because they don't have the emotional strength to be with a person with dementia. In addition, old family dynamics come into play and make caregiving impossible for them. While it's difficult to do, allowing each family member to have their relationship and way of supporting your loved one and accepting it as their best, will help you keep your family intact.

Keep looking for the contributions that each family member does make, and not what they don't do. If possible, have lots of communication. I met a wonderful caregiver who texts a report to her siblings after every visit with her Mom. Her brother isn't able to help the way she and her sister do. They accept what he can give, let go of the small stuff and focus on the big picture. They have committed that their family's long-term happiness is most important. Having good relationships with each other after all of the care is in the past is most important. If sibling relationships are strained, do your best to mend the fences and make sure your immediate family: you, your spouse and kids, stays strong.

Now is the time to adjust your expectations of yourself and others, especially with your siblings. It's time to have compassion not just for your loved one with dementia but for others in your family who aren't as strong as you, or who show their love in a way that is different from you. Find a place to vent. So many family caregivers end up with struggle in their family relationships because of conflict in how their loved one is being cared for. Do what you can to avoid this.

Create a plan with family members now so that family peace can be maintained. Do your best and know that other family members are doing their best, too.

BRINGING IN HELP

If you decide to bring in outside help, use the previous chapter. Make sure you find someone trained to care for a person with dementia. Make sure they are part of the ILOP (I Love Old People) club. Make sure they will respect your loved one and your family values. You're going to have to pay your caregiver a fair wage. This may vary from state to state and from city to city. There are agencies that provide caregivers, but the caregiver is paid far less than what you pay the agency. Caregiving, especially for a person with dementia, is not an easy job. It requires profound patience, deep compassion and a playful spirit. It also requires high emotional intelligence to see through the behavior to the feeling or struggle behind it. If you find someone you like, do all you can to hang on to him or her. Finding a compassionate family friend and having them trained can be a good way to go: someone your loved one knows and who knows your loved one. I've heard of and experienced the great joy caregivers develop for their clients, who become loved ones. There are stories of shared activities, going to theatre or even traveling together. It's a deeply satis-fying experience to bring that connection and joy to a person with dementia.

Having been on both sides of this situation, as a professional caregiver and also a family caregiver for my Mom and brother, I can see the benefit of looking for the best in each family member and also having outside help. When I'm with my mom, my tendency is to be less patient with her, to expect more of her. It's an old dynamic, and I see it! It is so frustrating that I am more frustrated with my own mother than I am with my clients.

ABUSE

This is a subject I wish we didn't have to discuss. We don't want to think about our elderly parents, who are losing so much of themselves and are so vulnerable, being exploited. I had this happen to a client and a family member. Both were taken advantage of by their caregivers. My client, Bea, was being manipulated by caregivers who were trying to get power of attorney taken from her family. The caregivers were slowly eroding her trust in her children, telling her that her children didn't care about her and were taking ad-vantage of her. A caregiver had gone as far as hiring a lawyer without the family's knowledge. When I met Bea, she was distraught, confused and depressed. She was angry and aggressive because of her heightened anxiety.

I felt like I was watching a disaster in slow motion. I went to Bea's daughter and told her what I knew. She, of course, quickly took the steps to ensure her mom's safety and discharge the people who were hurting her.

A similar thing happened to my elderly cousin. He brought in a caregiver when he was quite ill and needed help with daily activities and physical care. She took control of his finances, spent his money and nearly had ownership of his home. My Mom was the one who advocated for him and spent countless hours with social workers and attorneys to straighten it all out.

Others report theft of medication and personal items which are bad, but are actually minor offenses in the bigger picture. Abuse in facilities, such as neglect and overmedicating, is more common and more severe. Background checks and fingerprinting will tell you about a person's history. Paying close attention to red flags will keep you alerted to dangerous or destructive behavior. Be mindful of caregivers who are disrespectful or isolate your loved one. Arguing with you, especially in front of your loved one, might be a sign that they are trying to undermine your relationship with your loved one. If your loved one is wary, suspicious or uncharacteristically angry with you, this could be a sign of abuse by a caregiver. Communication with those close to you and your loved one will help you identify any changes. Vigilant attention to their finances will also safeguard you. Contracts with caregivers as to what are, and are not, their responsibilities will also put them on notice as to your expectations and your awareness of important matters.

PROBLEM SOLVING

If your loved one has sensitivities, let them be the guide in their solution. I knew a caregiver whose client was very sensitive to the clanging sounds in the kitchen when the dishes were being washed or put away. One solution is to have her leave the room while the kitchen was being cleaned up. But her client came up with the brilliant solution.

"We're going plastic."

They bought plastic reusable bowls, cups, and even cutlery! Yes, the plastic knives were less efficient, but the client was so happy to have come up with the solution and was able to stay in the kitchen after meals and help clear the dishes.

Another smart caregiver began using language early on that supported her father as he declined. He had some physical limitations early on so when he got up from a chair, she would repeat, "Left, right. Left, right," so that he would move his feet. This became a long-term memory for him and even as his memory declined, he was able to continue to understand what that means and move his feet to get from one place to the next. Finding language that can be repeated and put into the memory early on will help you as the years go on.

As the years go on...

This is going to be a long-term project, caring for your loved one with dementia. Some days, I feel like the day never ends and some days the time flies because we're in a flow and just enjoying being together. Watching a loved one change will hurt your heart. It takes a little while to get used to the new normal. But once expectations are adjusted, things roll along again. Look for the little gifts each time you spend with your loved one and let that carry you through the hard times.

CHAPTER 11

Abundant Lessons

Although I spent many years as a caregiver, professionally and personally, I had never experienced someone transforming in front of my eyes because of communication. Kerry taught me the value of compassion, communication and connection.

I went from being scared and unsure to being confident and happy. Because of that, I chose the path of being a caregiver and it has been a blessing. I have never done work that was so meaningful and powerful.

It isn't easy being a caregiver and when I meet others, especially family caregivers, I am once again inspired by the power of their commitment to their families and loved ones. I'm inspired by the patience and love that continues to grow as the memory fades.

When I think of Kerry, things have changed so much for her. She was on the fast track to financial success and power, even considering a career in politics. Then everything changed for her in a heartbeat. As she slipped away from her expensive clothes, slender body and influential friends, what was left was relationships. The people who are there for her day-to-day: the servers in the dining room where she lives, her devoted family, her attentive caregivers and a select few friends from childhood. It's that love which brings meaning and vitality to her now. It's a different life but there is still life. There is a lot of humor and play and joy that Kerry experiences each day because of the people in her life. She feels love and safety, validation and connection and she is present in the moment.

For me, the journey has been in knowing her. Really knowing her: her fears, her humor, her language, her idiosyncrasies. I had come to know just how she liked the car to be when I drove her to tennis, how many packs of tissues to bring and making sure we had sunscreen. It was my mission to make her day the best day it could be. When I succeeded, I felt great. When we had trouble, I got help and advice and implemented what I learned. When I saw her change based on those techniques, I was thrilled. I knew that others having struggles with their loved ones with dementia could benefit from my trials and the techniques I used.

My clients have made my life richer. I love to bring joy into their lives and ease to their families. There is a deep sense of satisfaction that I've felt by being of service to them. I've met with many families who have success by using the techniques outlined in these pages and have brought joy and peace to those who take on using them. These techniques are really about love. They work with our children, spouses and workmates. They create connection and respect and affinity.

Maybe someday there will be a cure for Alzheimer's disease. Maybe the trials and all the resources going toward finding a cure will pay off. There are certainly great minds working tirelessly in search of one. There are entire communities in Europe being designed to accommodate people with dementia called "dementia villages." This movement allows people with dementia to be who they are now. Instead of pushing an old reality on them, it supports their NEW reality. They are free to participate in regular activities like cooking and cleaning and have support to do so. There is less agitation and less need for medication in these villages. Wandering and exploring are safe and encouraged. We are at a pivotal time in dementia care. The first steps to take are in how we talk to people with dementia. Talk IS care. To learn to appreciate their new reality, even the childish or repetitive behavior, is the beginning toward access to better care and peace for them.

ABOUT MARISA PASQUINI

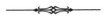

Marisa Pasquini is a speaker, bestselling author, and dementia expert. She trains professional and family caregivers of people with dementia using proven techniques that master upset and create peace.

Marisa brings 20 years of professional experience with organizations serving the elderly, people with intellectual disabilities, addictions, special needs, dementia and Alzheimer's. A former director of a nonprofit hospice agency, Marisa is the founder of the National Home Care Academy which provides training programs for professional and family caregivers.

Marisa's mission is to change the way people think about dementia - to replace fear and prejudice with education and compassion. She loves to brainstorm with families, agencies and caregivers, to help them solve their biggest challenges, create positive outcomes and joy (yes, JOY!) for caregivers, families, and people with dementia.

ACKNOWLEDGEMENTS

Thank you to Cory Sherman, I treasure our times working together. Thank you, Ernesto Paredes and Donna Barranco-Fisher for seeing something in me that moved me forward.

To my Activator, Melodee Meyer, whose shoulder continually nudges me forward on this fantastic voyage.

For all my loved ones with special needs and dementia.

You are the teachers.

To my partner, Jack Rief, who listens to my stories and put up with earlier and earlier wake-up calls so I could get this book written. Thank you for your gift of patience and keeping me nourished with delicious food.

Thanks to my parents, siblings and extended family for the early lessons on caring for a family member with special needs. Thank you for being pioneers in inclusion and making Rick one of the gang.

Thank you, Rick, for your special abilities and love. I'll always be your baby sister and you can keep me!

Thank you to Steve Najarro, Sage Parker, Johnny Miller and Randy Reid for the encouragement, brainstorming, and midnight texts.

You are the REAL DEAL!

Most of all, thank you caregivers who contribute to my growth and development. Without you, many would be lost. Thank you for doing the sometimes thankless job of caring for a person with dementia. You give from your hearts everyday and make a difference just by showing up.

BOOK MARISA TO SPEAK AT YOUR NEXT EVENT

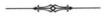

A transformative speaker, Marisa Pasquini has inspired large and small groups for many years. She educates and illuminates her audience by teaching techniques that master upset and create peace for people with dementia and their caregivers.

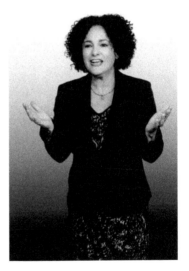

Dementia is an issue that affects so many people and it is her mission to erase the prejudice about dementia. She teaches new skills to help caregivers confidently and compassionately handle the challenges of caring for a person with dementia, and do it with confidence and joy.

Marisa brings 20 years serving the elderly, disabled and those with dementia and Alzheimer's. Her personal journey includes growing up with a brother with intellectual disabilities, as well as caring for her mother after a debilitating stroke.

To book Marisa as a speaker at your next event, meeting or conference find her at:

www.nationalhomecareacademy.com

DEMENTIA CARE MASTERY

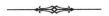

Most of us caring for a person with dementia are in a whole new world. The person in our care changes daily. There can be aggression, confusion, and anxiety. Not only do their behaviors vary from day to day but their triggers fluctuate, too. Add to it that most people caring for a person with dementia aren't trained to deal with the challenging emotions and behaviors. We all want to provide exceptional care with kindness and compassion. Training really can help.

The National Home Care Academy provides several training programs to help the family and professional caregiver maintain their joy while confidently navigating the challenges of caring for a person (or persons) with dementia.

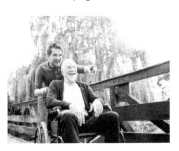

For more information, go to:

www.nationalhomecareacademy.com